I0478589

CODE FROM HOME

CODE FROM HOME

LAUNCH YOUR HOME-BASED MEDICAL BILLING SERVICE

Sandra L. Kocsis

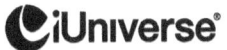

CODE FROM HOME
LAUNCH YOUR HOME-BASED MEDICAL BILLING SERVICE

Copyright © 2014 Sandra L. Kocsis.

All rights reserved. No part of this book may be used or reproduced by any means, graphic, electronic, or mechanical, including photocopying, recording, taping or by any information storage retrieval system without the written permission of the publisher except in the case of brief quotations embodied in critical articles and reviews.

The information contained in this book came from Sandra L. Kocsis and is believed to be accurate and up-to-date. However, neither the publisher nor the author guarantee the sources and reliability.

Neither the publisher nor the author shall be responsible for any exclusions, errors, or reparations stemming from the use of this information. The production is published with the understanding that the publisher and the author are supplying knowledge but are not attempting to provide business consulting or other trained services. If such services are required, the assistance of the appropriate professional should be sought.

iUniverse books may be ordered through booksellers or by contacting:

iUniverse
1663 Liberty Drive
Bloomington, IN 47403
www.iuniverse.com
1-800-Authors (1-800-288-4677)

Because of the dynamic nature of the Internet, any web addresses or links contained in this book may have changed since publication and may no longer be valid. The views expressed in this work are solely those of the author and do not necessarily reflect the views of the publisher, and the publisher hereby disclaims any responsibility for them.

Any people depicted in stock imagery provided by Thinkstock are models, and such images are being used for illustrative purposes only. Certain stock imagery © Thinkstock.

ISBN: 978-1-4917-4688-2 (sc)
ISBN: 978-1-4917-4691-2 (e)

Library of Congress Control Number: 2014916695

Printed in the United States of America.

iUniverse rev. date: 10/06/2014

Dedication

Along the way, I have gained insight from many professionals, colleagues, family, and friends. Some of the names that I would like to mention are my daughters, Ashley, Danielle, and Amy for showing their support and giving me unconditional love. I would like to thank Sid L. for always pushing me toward success and being supportive, even during the tough times. I would like to thank my mom, Pam L., for believing in me when no one else did and for helping me buy my first computer. I would like to mention my brother Ron R. and sister Katherine R. for keeping me on my toes. I would like to mention Ralf L. for having the courage and patience to hire, train, and encourage me to achieve successes that seemed unreachable, and for correcting errors in my proposal and billing letters. I would like to thank Carolyn F. and Sue C. for always being there and encouraging me to be my best self, as well as laughing and crying with me when life threw me curve balls. I would like to thank Dr. Stephen C. for being so patient with me while I learned medical terminology and the orthopedic process. I would like to thank American River College, California State University of Sacramento, Folsom Lake College, and Excelsior College for allowing me to persevere. Without all of you and the experiences I have gained I may have ended on a different path.

Table of Contents

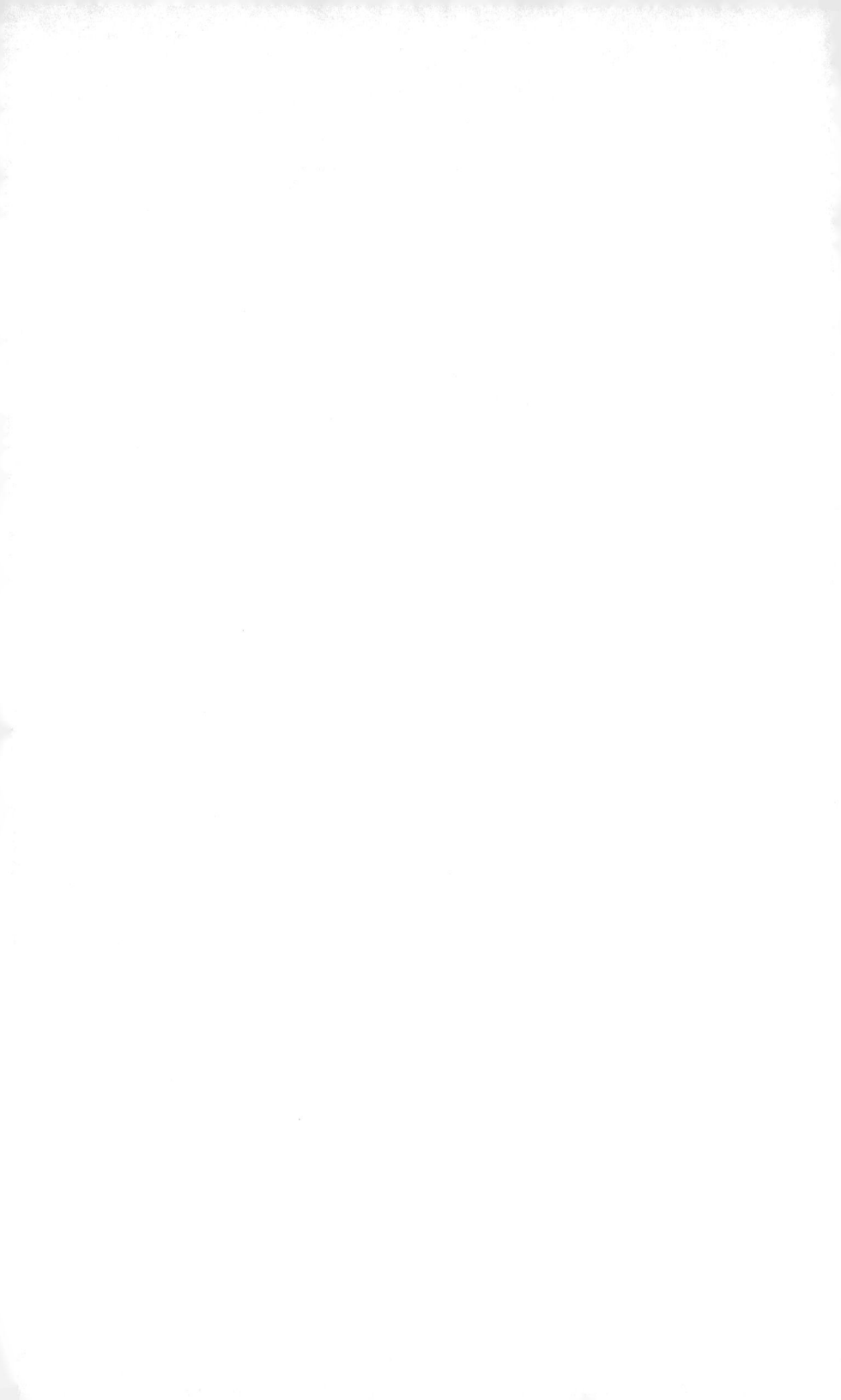

Introduction

Think of working for yourself and avoiding the hustle and bustle of traffic. What about avoiding the pressure and the time it takes to get to an employer in order to punch in on time? Consider dodging the boss, who wants everything done his or her way and never considers the ideas of others. Take into account the constant compromising with coworkers. Imagine never dealing with the rules and regulations that must be followed while working for someone else. Now the ball is in your court. It is up to you. You can start your own business. What is more, it is a business you can start with very modest expenditure, although as the volume of your business grows, you may be surprised at how easily and naturally you invest in new equipment and new technology to improve your productivity and, of course, your income. Earning your own income comes with responsibility, and everything you need to know to get started is included in this book. It starts with understanding and building up for the marketing phase. Then there's the nuts and bolts of the business: diagnosis and procedural coding, verifying reimbursement eligibility, and obtaining the information necessary for home-based medical billing. There is a sample proposal for soliciting business from physicians and sample billing and collection letters that will make solving many patient situations easy. Along the way, I relate experiences that help explain the processes. Finally, there is preparing for month-end obligations that will give clients a sense of how well this process is working for them. A saying I have learned to accept in this ever-changing field is "Embrace change." Trends among insurance carriers and physicians' offices that are current as I write this may be different at the time you start your business. HMOs (health maintenance organizations), PPOs (preferred provider organizations), EPOs (exclusive provider organizations), and IPAs (independent practice associations) all handle their billing differently. The HCPCS

(Healthcare Common Procedural Coding System), Medicare, Medicaid/Medi-Cal, worker's compensation, Champus, and other services and systems regularly change their billing rules. Physicians receive updates about these changes. An important part of your job will be to stay current by reading these updates and contacting insurance companies and services about any questions you have. Attending seminars, participating in workshops, or going online and doing research are necessary. Medicare and Medicaid create provider manuals that can be obtained through the Center for Medicare & Medicaid Services Web site. (For current URLs and additional information on the resources I reference, please turn to the Additional Resources page at the end of the book.) Every insurance company provides information to help you submit accurate, high-quality bills according to their guidelines. It is vital to your business that you receive the most complete and accurate medical billing information in order to avoid having claims denied for reimbursement. This includes the regulations of the Affordable Care Act. Health insurance is the most common way that patients are able to pay for their health care costs. Physicians will probably not want to become involved with increased regulations for decreased reimbursements. This also guarantees that someone will need to do the billing in order for the doctor to get paid. Remember, you need to convince those doctors that you can take away the concern of all of that administrative side of their practice, in order for them to concentrate on providing great patient care. The United States has set out on a journey to deliver the highest quality patient care in an affordable way. Whether the health care is delivered in a clinical setting, office, or hospital, delivering high-quality care as efficiently as possible has become very important. Meanwhile, there have been legal maneuverings and congressional debate about the future of health care reform. As the reform has been implemented, government reimbursement rates have been cut, while demands have increased for doctors and hospitals to deliver more care for less money. The challenge that most health care providers and facilities must face is how to continue serving growing numbers of government-sponsored patients at a cost close to what Medicare insurance pays them. As doctors and hospitals seek solutions to their financial challenges, they are also creating new opportunities to better serve their patients. This means that doctors and hospitals need to remain open to different approaches to delivering their services and providing patients with a level of personal care they can't get anywhere else. If doctors and hospitals can achieve this goal, then they'll be able to grow while maintaining a stable and secure health care force. What this means is that ways of billing for services must follow these changes. Adjustments must continuously be made to ensure medical services receive the maximum reimbursement possible in a timely manner.

Part One

MARKETING YOURSELF

CHAPTER 1
Are You Interested?

If you love the phrase "independent businessman or businesswoman" but are afraid of the responsibilities and hard work, don't be. The responsibilities are minimal, and the work can be easy if there's a system in place. A system is, from the first step to the last step, a process of working that you have created and feel comfortable with. This book is going to help you develop a system.

Having your own business at home means you are your own boss. You must keep your commitments and meet your deadlines. If you can do that, you are on your way to success.

Within reason, home medical billing is something anyone can get into. If you can read, write, do math, use a phone, communicate, and use a keyboard, then you have the basic skills required to proceed. Ten-key calculator skills are also useful. After that, it is up to you what you are willing to put into it in order to build a business that you are satisfied with and that brings in an income that satisfies you.

If you are wondering whether you can do this, let me reassure you that you can. People in this field come from many types of backgrounds. Some have taken a medical billing and collections course or have worked for a medical billing service. Some have worked in a hospital or physician's office. Some have never worked in medical billing or taken a course in it.

Whatever your background, there is always a need to learn and grow, and this is true for a medical billing career. There are a wealth of classes that can be taken to become a certified medical biller, but certification is not necessary. The American Medical Association or local colleges can help you get started if you want to seek certification.

The resources provided in this book will help you get started in learning medical billing and collections from the ground up. With some persistence, you can learn everything you need to know. You will get the rest through your own working experience. Once you have learned how to submit a claim form, following up will teach you what the payers need and how they want to receive it from you in order to get the claims paid.

The proposal, patient, insurance, and collection letters in this book were developed based on my own experience and working knowledge, with input from professionals out in the field. I have used these letters time and time again, and they have proven very effective. The letters will help resolve any issues that may prevent the payer from paying the claims.

As you begin learning and pursuing your own home-based medical billing service, you will see how easily you can move through the tasks, one at a time, until you have conquered what it takes to be your own successful boss.

When starting your own business, there are several things to think about. You should investigate any licensing or registration requirements that are in effect where you live.

One of the first things to decide is what to call your business. If you name your business after yourself, it is not necessary to file a fictitious name statement (also called a DBA, or "doing business as" statement). If you are planning on calling your business something other than your own legal name, you may need to file a fictitious name statement. You may also be required to advertise your business in the local newspaper or other source by the clerk-recorder's office. Your county's clerk-recorder's office will provide any necessary paperwork for you to fill out and submit with a small payment. In my county, the cost was $30.00. To be sure, contact the small business administration online at http://www.sba.gov/, and they will be able to help you narrow down the search for the area that you are in.

Next, you may need a business license. If so, your county will provide the application. In my county, the cost was $108. They also provided some stipulations for operating a home-based business, including:

- There shall be no exterior display or evidence of home occupation.
- A home occupation shall be conducted only within an enclosed living area of the dwelling, detached accessory structure that does not exceed any size limitation contained elsewhere in this ordinance, or attached garage, or, in the case of a garage/yard sale or plant nursery, adjacent to a dwelling or a garage.
- Home occupations shall not be permitted out-of-doors on the property or in any trailer or temporary structure unless allowed by subsection or unless otherwise consistent with this chapter.
- No mechanical equipment shall be used that creates visible or audible interference in line voltage outside the dwelling or unit that creates noise, odor, glare, smoke, or dust not normally associated with residential uses.
- No commercial vehicles, including taxis and limousines, shall be stored on the site, even if owned, rented, or leased by the home occupation operator, unless allowed pursuant to the provisions.
- No more than one commercial vehicle round trip per day, not including taxis or limousine trips, shall be made for the purpose of picking up or delivering raw materials, finished products, equipment, or similar materials to or from the home occupation residence.

- One employee, other than actual residents of the dwelling, may be engaged in the home occupation when operated from a single-family detached home.
- No home occupation or combination of home occupations on a single site shall involve more than three patrons visiting the site at any one time and a maximum of fifteen patrons per day except for occasional garage/yard sales.
- Home occupations shall be conducted primarily between 7:00 a.m. and 10:00 p.m.

More information about the stipulations of owning a home-based business can be found at your county's clerk-recorder's office. General information can be obtained from a reference librarian. A professional accountant will help you make a checklist of important information that may be necessary to grow your business. Another great resource is the Small Business Administration, who can help solve the questions that may come up as you read and encounter situations. Their website has a small business planner, services, tools, and local resources that may be helpful.

After that, you will need to obtain a tax identification number from the Internal Revenue Service. There are guidelines for paying taxes and rules for what constitutes the ability to "write off" certain items on your taxes. You will want to know what you can write off and what you can't as you make decisions about investing in your business—for example, the consequences of leasing versus purchasing equipment, or inviting a client to lunch.

Think about whether you will be a sole proprietor, LLC (limited liability company), or something else. Talking with an accountant can help you understand the differences.

Finally, you will need to think about how you are going to market yourself in order to obtain clients. Think about your communication ability, business skills, experience, and service proposal.

CHAPTER 2
Communications

Personal presence is a powerful quality that displays charisma, character, and leadership skills. Three important qualities of personal presence include professional appearance, verbal communication, and a self-confident demeanor. Often people use these characteristics without giving them much thought. Putting more thought into them can help you develop in a way that will make you stand out in a room full of people.

One of the most valuable tools for personal and professional success is good verbal communication. Vocal effectiveness supports word choices and voice tones that send the intended message out correctly. Some communications coaches refer to the acronym KISS (keep it short and simple) when teaching vocal effectiveness. The same words can mean different things to different people, so it's important to choose words that both the sender and receiver will readily understand.

Be yourself. When you speak, do not suddenly try to use big words and long sentences to impress the receiver. If you do, you will probably miscommunicate and sound silly or at least stiff and pretentious. Stick to facts. Offer your opinion only when you feel it is appropriate.

Be courteous and keep to the point. Being too short can seem rude, but a wordy, rambling talker wastes the receiver's time.

Be complete. Make sure that you include all pertinent information.

Avoid jargon. Jargon is specialized, technical language not normally used in everyday communication. For example, if you were coding breast implants, you would not refer to them as "boobs," during a professional conversation. Using appropriate medical terminology keeps the conversation professional. You should avoid such terms unless you are certain the receiver will understand them.

Miscommunication occurs when something goes wrong between the sender and the receiver. Be sure to speak clearly, listen closely, read thoroughly, and watch gestures and facial expressions to help avoid miscommunication.

Communication starts with word choices. In the book *Essentials of Business Communication*, author Mary Ellen Guffey states, "Think twice about sprinkling your conversation with like, you know, and up talk (making declarative sentences sound like questions). You don't want to send the wrong message with unwitting and unprofessional behavior" (2009, p. 5). The words you choose demonstrates how knowledgeable you are about the subject you are talking about.

Be aware of whom you can joke with and whom you cannot. One person might think your joke is funny and another person might think your joke is disrespectful. Humor at work makes work more fun, but always remember that you are in a professional environment.

Your attitude plays a part in your professional presence. When you are at work, it is best to leave personal problems outside. A happy and positive attitude can radiate to others and make the working environment more enjoyable.

One of the most essential aspects of a professional presence is projecting a self-confident demeanor. Traits that contribute to a self-confident demeanor include making eye contact with whoever you're talking to; having good posture and standing up straight but not allowing your posture to become ramrod rigid; greeting a new person with a firm but not too strong handshake; speaking clearly; not mumbling or hesitating; listening attentively when others are speaking; maintaining a positive, can-do attitude; and being polite and respectful to those you meet or work with. I could go on and on, because there are a lot of aspects to this one characteristic!

Challenges to maintaining a self-confident demeanor can include feeling insecure about your ability to do a new task. You need to remind yourself that you can do it and perhaps work a little harder to master a new skill to bring your self-confidence back.

Another challenge is knowing your area of expertise. There are many people who can look and act a part, but there is no substance to them when the challenge calls for action. On the other hand, a person may be shy but very able. This capable individual can find it very difficult to portray a professional attitude. Practicing communication only gets her or him so far, but once she or he is in the door, her or his work speaks volumes. One solution is to develop a personal support network that will provide ongoing, positive feedback and more opportunity to practice the professional presence in front of an encouraging audience.

CHAPTER 3
Selling Your Skills

In order to sell your skills, you need to establish what they are. The first and most important thing to realize is that speed is secondary to accuracy. If you transpose numbers or submit misspellings and errors, insurance companies will deny charges and physicians may develop doubts. This will lower your standing in the eyes of potential clients, as well as reduce your income.

Knowledge of the computer keyboard and 10-key calculator is recommended. Having secretarial skills and experience are a plus, but not a must. When it comes down to it, it's not your skills or your experience that gets you your client. It is how well you get along with your client and whether you are able to build trust that determines whether that client will risk his or her income by relying on you. Your skills and experience will be appreciated as part of how you successfully implement your working system and carry out the duties described in your service proposal.

The medical and legal records that you will read and fill out are not much different from the academic records you filled out in school. As long as you follow directions and proofread, you're safe.

The reference books you'll need are as easy to use as a dictionary. As long as you read word for word until you understand, you can't go wrong.

No one is likely to be an expert at all things. Confidence and a willingness to learn are what you need to convey.

The following worksheet will help you assess where you stand with the skills that are relevant to the medical billing field. Rate yourself as honestly as possible.

Skill and Experience List

1 = No skill or experience
2 = Slight experience and some skill
3 = Average skill or experience
4 = Better-than-average skill or experience
5 = Expert

Circle one number for each category:

Accuracy	1 2 3 4 5
Typing	1 2 3 4 5
10-key calculator	1 2 3 4 5
Shorthand	1 2 3 4 5
Filing	1 2 3 4 5
Data entry	1 2 3 4 5
Word processing	1 2 3 4 5
Accounts payable	1 2 3 4 5
Accounts receivable	1 2 3 4 5
Medical terminology	1 2 3 4 5
Procedure coding	1 2 3 4 5
Diagnosis coding	1 2 3 4 5
Medicare guidelines	1 2 3 4 5
Medicaid or Medi-Cal guidelines	1 2 3 4 5
Worker's compensation guidelines	1 2 3 4 5
Commercial insurance	1 2 3 4 5
Health maintenance organization (HMO)	1 2 3 4 5
Preferred provider organization (PPO)	1 2 3 4 5
Exclusive provider organization (EPO)	1 2 3 4 5

Collections	1 2 3 4 5
Self-organization	1 2 3 4 5
Other_____	1 2 3 4 5

Looking back at what you circled, you now know which areas you are good at and which areas need to be improved upon. Take on one task at a time, and you will be closer to reaching your goals.

CHAPTER 4
Letter Writing

Letter writing is a common means to communicate and is widely used in this business. However, what we learned in school doesn't always stay with us. In order to get your message across, it is important to refresh your letter-writing skills.

One of the best places to refresh your writing skills is at the Purdue Online Writing Lab (OWL). Here, you can navigate through the areas you feel need work. The following is an outline of some of the items you may need to review.

A. Punctuation

1. . = period: needed to stop sentences.
2. ? = question mark: asks a question.
3. , = comma: tells the reader to pause and then go on.
   a. The most common use is to separate words in a series.
   Example: I like to eat fruits, vegetables, meat, and cheese.
   b. When speaking directly to a person or a group, you separate that person or group from the rest of the sentence with commas.
   Example: "Excuse me, Mr. Dragon, but your foot is in the backseat of my car."
   c. Phrases in a series are also separated by commas.
   Example: The town where the dragon lived was known for its rainbow-colored rose bushes, backyards full of tree houses, front yards full of grass, restaurant that sold fried bathtub rings, and perfectly terrible jail.
   d. Use a comma before the words *and, but, for, or,* and *nor* when they connect two independent parts of a

sentence. Don't use a comma before those words when the second part of the sentence can't stand alone.

Example: The dragon was sorry about ruining the mayor's new car, but he was not willing to replace it. (*He was not willing to replace it* stands alone.)

The dragon was sorry about the mayor's new car but was unwilling to replace it. (*Was unwilling to replace it* cannot stand alone.)

e. When one part of a sentence introduces another part, a comma may be needed to make the meaning clear.

Example: If the mayor had been riding a bicycle, the dragon might not have stepped on it.

f. A phrase that adds information about the subject of the sentence is often set off with commas.

Example: The dragon, who had stopped on many cars, always avoided destroying bicycles.

g. A phrase that says something so important about the subject that the sentence wouldn't make sense or would be inaccurate without it is not set off with commas.

Example: Dragons who step on cars must pay a fine or go to jail. (If you took out *who step on cars*, you would get *Dragons must pay a fine or go to jail*, which is not true.)

h. Place a comma after the greeting of a friendly or informal letter, between the date and the year, between a city and a state, and after *yes* or *no* when talking to someone.

4. ; = semicolon: joins two sentences that are so closely related they should not be separated by a period.

Example: Old age made the dragon wise; travel made him witty. (The semicolon could be replaced with *and* or a period.)

—You can't use a semicolon to join two parts of a sentence that can't stand alone.

5. : = colon: stops readers just long enough to let them know they're in for a long list. Don't use in a short list.

   —Colons are used to join two related sentences, but they are used only when the second part of the sentence explains, expands, or illustrates the first part.

6. " " = quotation marks: used whenever a writer borrows words that belong to someone else.

   —A period or comma almost always goes inside the second quotation mark.

B. Elements of a Business Letter

Full Block Form
All lines are typed flush with the left margin, including the date and complimentary close.

Paragraphs
Paragraphs are indicated by double-line spacing or triple-line spacing when the letter has been double-spaced already.

Letterhead
Choose quality paper with quality printing.

Date Line
The horizontal placement is flush left and should always follow these rules:

1. Type the date line fourteen to sixteen lines down from the top of the page.
2. Spell the name of the month in full.
3. Do not use "nd," "st," "th," or "rd" after the day of the month. (Correct: June 1, 1950. Incorrect: June 1st, 1950.)
4. The date of the month is separated from the year by a comma.

Inside Address
The inside address must match the address on the envelope. Begin on the sixth line down from the date line.

Attention Line
This is an extension of the inside address and is used when you wish to make sure a particular individual or department receives the letter.

Salutation
Place the salutation below the inside address (or the attention line, if there is one) and above the body of the letter. It is blocked at the left margin with two spaces above it and below it.

Subject Line
If there is a subject line, type it on the second line below the salutation. It may be started flush at the left margin or centered. The word *subject* or *regarding* or *re*, followed by a colon, is placed before the description of the subject matter.

Body of the Letter
The primary purpose of your letter should be clear from the start. The message should be arranged so that key features, such as points to be emphasized, date provided, and action recommended will be favorably taken by the reader. Remember to create a new paragraph when the idea changes or when emphasis is necessary.

Complimentary Close
This is the simple phrase that concludes your conversation with the reader. Only the initial word is capitalized. It is followed by a comma. It is typed in alignment with the signature line and the date line. Frequently used closes include "Yours very truly," "Very truly yours," and "Sincerely."

Dictator's Identification and Signature

You should type the dictator's name and title immediately below the space for his or her signature. Depending upon the size of the handwriting, leave as few as three to as many as six blank lines to allow room for the signature to fit easily between the complimentary close and his or her typed name and title.

Reference Initials

These are the initials of the person who dictated and the person who typed the letter. The dictator's initials should be typed in capital letters, followed by a slash, followed by the typist's initials in lowercase letters, with no spaces between these parts. The initials should look like this: JLL/ssk. Type the reference initials two spaces below the dictator's typed name.

Enclosure Notation

If there is an enclosure, a notation is made below the reference initials. It is typed flush with the left margin. If there is one enclosure, *enc* should be used to indicate it. If there is more than one enclosure, the number of enclosures should be indicated by a number in parentheses: enc (2).

Copy Notation

A letter addressed to one person may be important to one or more other individuals. If this is the case, copies of the original letter may be sent to other individuals. These carbon copies should be noted by *cc* followed by a colon, then the party's name: cc: John Smith

Postscript

A postscript is an afterthought that is added to the letter after it has been dictated or typed. It is rarely used in business letters, but everyone needs to be familiar with it. The abbreviation P.S. is used to identify the postscript. It is typed two lines below the last notation that is in the letter. It is typed flush with the left margin.

Second Page Headings

If the letter requires one or more continuation pages, the heading of the second and subsequent pages must contain three bits of information: the name of the addressee, the page number, and the date. Two accepted forms for this headings are:

I.G. Bright, MD   -2-   March 4, 2009

or

    I. G. Bright, MD
    Page 2
    March 4, 2009

Letter writing is a useful tool because it is a very common method of communication. Convey your professionalism through proper formatting and word choices, in order for your message to be perceived the way it was intended.

CHAPTER 5

Proposing

Proposing is the formal term for putting forth your intention and the plan that you want to be considered. Here is an example of a service proposal for medical billing. This proposal is not intended for you to copy but as a pattern or tool to help you develop your own. A proposal should reflect your communication style and unique skills.

> Dear Doctor,
>
> It is my intention to eliminate concern whether or not you, as a physician, will get your well-deserved income for services rendered. What about decreasing the time and expense it takes to complete the tasks required to obtain your income? I am prepared to take the worry of your accounts receivable away!
>
> My interest is to fulfill your goal by doing what I do best: medical billing and collecting, at a rate of only_____. [Note to reader: I used the figure of 7 percent of gross receipts. You should research an appropriate rate for your area, as described in chapter 21.] I have the equipment to submit your charges quickly and accurately, and you'll receive reimbursement rapidly.
>
> My experience includes teaching medical reception, insurance billing, collections, and transcription at our local college, as well as

personally working in doctors' offices. Through teaching and several years' experience, I have learned to focus on accuracy. It is important that everyone involved receive the most complete information to avoid delay.

It's simple. On a weekly basis, I will obtain from you the patients' demographic information, copies of any insurance information, procedures performed, diagnoses, and fees. I will verify the insurance benefits, code all of the procedures and diagnoses, and submit the charges to the insurance companies in a timely manner.

Upon receiving payment, I will deposit funds directly into your bank account, either weekly or according to a process you negotiate. Follow-up will be done not less than every thirty days: first on the date I receive the charge, and then at the end of every month thereafter. I have prepared collection letters that have proven effective with both patients and insurance companies.

Within ten days after your month-end closing, you will receive a general ledger report that will contain all of the charges billed, the payment adjustments, and the amount of payments deposited during the month. You will also receive a computer-generated report of your total accounts receivable that will tell you how each account is aging. At that time, I will prepare your statement based on_____. [Note to reader: the same rate that you quoted in the second paragraph would be restated here.]

I believe you will achieve your goal of receiving the maximum reimbursement without spending the time you could be spending with your patients.

Please take one minute to call me for additional information.

Sincerely yours,

The proposal should be printed on your personal letterhead using high-quality paper. Paper retailers can advise you regarding the best quality paper.

In addition to sending proposal letters such as this, you will want to market yourself in other ways. Decide how you want to advertise and get the word out.

I wanted to gain interest and entice everyone to read my proposal. Considering how physicians like the look of a diploma, I printed my proposals, rolled them up, and tied them with a red bow to resemble a diploma.

Then I thought about the fastest way to get my proposal out there. I thought about going to parking lots and putting them on peoples' vehicle windows. I thought about mailing them to every physician in the Yellow Pages. I decided that the fastest way to reach many physicians was to go to the hospitals and put them in their mail/communication boxes.

Let me share the details of my experience with this. I called a hospital to obtain permission to put my proposals in the doctors' boxes, and they granted it to me. After placing the proposals in their boxes, I went home. Several hours later, I had a nursing supervisor call me to say that I wasn't allowed to put them there and that I needed to come back and pick them up. I explained that I had obtained permission and from whom I obtained that permission, but she still made me go get them. Frustrated and embarrassed, I went back to that hospital and picked them up. Before I picked them all up, however, one physician read the proposal and called me for an interview. He became my first client.

Marketing can take time. All I can say is never give up. Someone will say yes.

CHAPTER 6
Interviewing

An interview is a personal conference or meeting during which you are questioned to determine whether or not your service proposal will be accepted by that business. Most people are familiar with job interviews for potential employees, but service providers are interviewed too.

Some of the questions that may be asked during your interview are:

Why you and not someone else?
What are your credentials?
What do you know about reimbursement rates?
How long will it take to obtain reimbursement for my services?
Have you ever done this before?
How successful have you been?

Having answers to these questions ready will help you succeed in the interview.

Your answers should be honest and portray confidence. For instance, to describe why they should hire you and not someone else, you could say that your rates are better than anyone else's because you have lower overhead costs. (Make sure you have done the research to back this up!) Plus, you focus on accuracy, which allows speed to come naturally. Convince them that you will be forthcoming and will operate in a very timely manner.

The question about your credentials can be answered by letting them know how your experience or knowledge will benefit their practice. Even if you do not have experience, after reading this book, you will have knowledge.

Before going on an interview, it is best to practice some billing with pretend patients, which will allow you to honestly answer yes, you have done this before. Having the confidence and the knowledge to face certain questions with appropriate answers will reveal to the interviewer that he or she should choose you over anyone else.

An interview may involve filling out an application. Here are some tips on completing an application:

1. Come prepared. Have a pen, sample application answers, and a list of three personal references with their addresses and phone numbers.
    a. Never ask for a pen or a phone book. If you do, this may suggest you are disorganized.
    b. Always inform your references that you will be using them as references.

2. Read instructions thoroughly.
    a. Always print legibly, unless another format is indicated.
    b. They are trying to find out if you can follow directions, not how well you can print.

3. Answer every question. If a question doesn't apply to you, acknowledge it with a dash (—) or with N/A for "not applicable." Don't leave the answer space blank. If you leave it blank, a reader might think you didn't understand the question or that, for some reason, you didn't wish to answer the question because you were hiding something.

4. For questions pertaining to injury:

    a. "Do you have any physical limitations that preclude you from performing all the duties of this position?" The proper answer to this should be no. If you can't physically do the job, then don't apply in the first place.

    b. "Have you had an industrial accident resulting in time loss?" If the answer to this is yes, then in the section marked "Give details," do *not* explain how the injury occurred. State that you have recovered and that you can physically handle this job. *Never* write "severe back injury," "slipped disc," or similar diagnoses. Write "muscle strain" or "back strain" instead. Stay away from the word *injury* and minimize use of medical terms, which may alarm the client.

    c. "Why did you leave your last job?" If you were laid off, indicate so. If you left because of industrial injury, state something like, "I was put out of commission for a while because I strained my back, but I am recovered." Or you can simply write, "Will discuss during the interview."

5. Be neat and check your spelling.

6. You may get an interview immediately after you have completed your application. If you are told the client will call you, ask when you might expect to hear or ask if you may follow up with a call in a few days.

A professional image builds trust and confidence in the interviewer. Not only should you look professional, but you should sound professional and write professionally. A company wants to know that a person it has hired is going to enhance the company's business, not bring it down.

The first impression is the most important part of the interview. That is the first personal contact that the company has with you, which is why it is best to do a great job the first time.

Doing a great job starts with appearance. When attending an interview, you should be clean, styled, modestly made up, wearing businesslike clothes, and using a light perfume/cologne or none at all.

Your well-written proposal, cover letter, and résumé should be with you to hand out again, just in case the interviewer has misplaced the one he or she originally received.

Speak clearly and concisely, with appropriate word choices. This tells the interviewer what level of professional he or she is dealing with.

All of this together presents enough information to the interviewer so that he or she will know that you are the type of person who will help the company grow.

An additional note about body language: body language shows unconscious information about how a person is feeling. Appropriate body language includes sitting up straight, arms relaxed at the side or gently in the lap, legs together on the floor or gently crossed in front, and facial expressions that are happy and calm.

Remember that most interviewers aren't accustomed to this situation either. Unless the interviewer works in human resources, he or she probably doesn't get a lot of experience doing interviews. Even if the interviewer is nervous, your body language can help to relax the situation.

Inappropriate body language includes slouching, folded arms, spread legs, and frowning facial expressions. This type of body language creates a tense environment. The point is to make the interview as pleasant as possible and that starts with body language.

Remember that first impressions are lasting ones. This is your chance to shine. Make the most of it, make a friend in the interview, and you will be the one the company chooses.

Chapter 7

Ethics

Ethics comprise a system of moral principles. Most of us know what's right and what's wrong. Ethics is more than just obeying the laws. You could behave legally and still not be ethical. In the book *Ethics in Health Administration*, Eileen E. Morrison states, "For example, if you are a hospital administrator in a large city, it might be acceptable for you to go to a bar after work and have a drink. In a small community, that same behavior might be seen as unethical, and even be reported to the Board of Trustees" (2011, p. 23). Sometimes behaving a certain way is perfectly acceptable in one context or with one group of people, but that same behavior comes across as unethical in another context or group.

Ethics comes down to you and how you behave. As a professional, you are ultimately the one who must choose the actions that you take. Start by thinking about the community in which you live. Be aware of the mission and values that you want to display. Thinking about your personal ethics will help you apply ethics to your daily decision making.

Personality

You must maintain a personality that's positive. A positive person:

—Develops an understanding of human relations
—Is sympathetic and kind
—Is courteous
—Is thoughtful
—Is pleasant and cheerful
—Is tactful

—Is honest
—Has self-confidence
—Has a sincere interest
—Leaves his or her personal problems at home
—Conducts him- or herself with dignity

Appearance

Your appearance should set a good example. Dressing like a professional is critical, especially in a health care facility. You represent the facility and your business. You are a representative for the patient and the doctors and nurses who are involved in patient care. If you are dressed shabbily, you will not get the respect you deserve.

Dress for the job and the respect that you want. Put some time into your grooming, within the limitations of any dress code and your budget. Too much makeup and long fingernails do not exhibit a professional image. Although most health care professionals have a specific dress code to adhere to, such as scrubs and lab jackets, that doesn't mean that you can't put yourself forward in a professional manner.

Improving professional presence takes understanding and a willingness to change. The first step is reading the dress code of the company you are planning on working in or are working for. Once you have an understanding of what the expectations about your appearance are, look around you and see how most people are presenting themselves. Learn from the people who have become successful and dress accordingly.

Responsibility

You are asking to assume responsibility for doctors' incomes. To prove you have the ability to do so will require:

—Careful planning of time, the doctors' and yours
—Confidentiality regarding the doctors' office procedures
—Cooperation with the doctors and the patients
—Loyalty
—Watching for ways to improve
—Considering the patients' comfort first
—Diplomacy in dealing with other people
—Acting as a public relations person for the doctors
—Refraining from making medical judgments
—Keeping all patient demographic information confidential unless it's necessary to collect a debt

Confidentiality

One of the worst business sins you can commit is failing to respect your clients' confidentiality. You will likely know a great deal about your clients' business, financial, and even personal affairs.

Of course, if you find that you are being asked to do things which go against your conscience, or if you merely wish no longer to work with a particular client, you are free to discontinue your association. If there is clear illegality, you might feel compelled to report it to the appropriate authorities. Even in this situation, however, you must maintain confidentiality when speaking to anyone other than the appropriate authorities.

You must never, ever gossip about your clients, either to your friends or other clients. If it is known that you cannot be trusted, your career will be negatively affected.

HIPAA

HIPAA stands for the Health Insurance Portability and Accountability Act, which is a set of federal guidelines that protect patients' privacy. HIPAA was enacted in 1996, and also includes provisions for administrative simplification. Everyone who works with patients and their medical records must adhere to HIPAA guidelines. Visit the Health and Human Services website to review all of the information needed to fully understand and comply with these guidelines.

CHAPTER 8
Cultural Competence

Cultural competence is being sensitive to cultures other than one's own. Cultural diversity in American society and our workplaces requires that we gain perception and an understanding of other peoples' beliefs, values, and backgrounds.

In the book, *Medical-Surgical Nursing* by Sharon Lewis, it tells us that cultural competence, "Involves an awareness and acceptance of cultural differences, self-awareness, knowledge of the client's culture, and adaptation of skills to meet the clients' needs" (2013, p. 25).

Good communication is important in how a client feels, encouraging him or her to share information about his or her culture. Good communication includes eye contact, listening, and controlling one's tone of voice. Knowing how different cultures perceive these aspects of communication will help build trust and make communication easier.

Cross-cultural appropriateness when dealing with a diverse population will give clients confidence that the management of their business comes from a place of understanding and consideration of others.

Part Two

THE BUSINESS OF CODING

CHAPTER 9
Coding

Physicians use a common language of names and terms (*nomenclature*) to communicate with the organizations that reimburse them for services rendered—primarily insurance companies and the government. Specific codes are recognized and accepted by most payers. These codes represent diagnoses, physician services and procedures, and medical services and supplies.

The medical billing representative's role in this process is to translate written diagnoses and procedures into numeric and alphanumeric codes, which communicate to the payers the reasons for providing the medical services being billed. To be fairly compensated, the physician and you need to understand and use these codes correctly.

One of the best ways to learn medical terminology is to look up terms that you are not familiar with in a medical dictionary. There are many respected medical dictionaries, including *Taber's Cyclopedic Medical Dictionary* and *Mosby's Dictionary of Medicine, Nursing & Health Professions*. The key is to have one in hand to refer to when terms are present that you do not understand.

CHAPTER 10

Diagnosis Coding

Some physicians have little or nothing to do with the coding system. Therefore, it is important that you know and stay updated on behalf of the physicians. You need to inform your clients of any changes that apply to their practices. Many physicians have preprinted forms that contain all of the procedure and diagnosis codes. The physicians usually check the box that applies to the patient you are billing for.

Insurance companies require a code to describe a patient's diagnosis. The physician must give you the diagnosis for every patient you will be billing for. You apply the correct code.

The code comes from a book called *International Classification of Diseases, Clinical Modification*, ninth or tenth edition, also known as ICD9 and ICD10. The American Medical Association is one of the best sources to get this book. Optum Coding is another place to buy it. This book is an essential part of medical billing. As of this writing, most offices still use ICD9, but since the ICD10 has been developed, they may be using this updated version. You need volumes 1 and 2 of the ICD, whichever edition you are using. Volume 1 is the numerical list, and volume 2 is the alphabetical index.

The best way to obtain knowledge about diagnosis coding is to read the instructions in the front of the ICD. Since you have to buy updates every year, immediately read about changes and apply them for the year you are billing in. The instructions are simple to understand, and the book contains exercises to help you determine the best code for a diagnosis description. A medical dictionary is a great tool to help you understand what you are coding.

Sometimes the physician will give you a code for the diagnosis. You need to double-check that the code is correct in order to avoid delay in processing the claim. If you submit a cancer code for an eye problem, then you, the physician, the patient, and the payer will be affected. Delay in reimbursement could happen. It is important to be accurate. Speed will come later.

To give you an idea of what you'll do when diagnosis coding, here is what a coding exercise looks like.

1. Use volume 2, the alphabetical index, to locate the main word of the diagnosis. The arrangement of the alphabetical index is by condition.

2. Read any note that appears under the main word.

3. Read any terms enclosed in parentheses following the main entry, as well as subterms under the main entry. Do not skip over any subterms while looking for the proper code.

    Example: The diagnosis is chronic alcoholic liver disease.
    Step 1. Look under *disease* (the condition) in volume 2.
    Step 2. Find *liver* in alphabetical order under *disease*.
    Step 3. Locate the subterm *alcoholic*.
    Step 4. Locate the second subterm *chronic*. The correct code is 571.3.

4. Refer to the numerical list, volume 1, to verify that the code number you have selected is in accord with the desired classification of the diagnosis. Never code directly from the alphabetical index because important instructions often appear only in the numerical list. Look

for exclusion notes, which refer to terms or conditions that are not included within the code and title under which the note appears. Exclusion notes will direct you to the correct code.

Example A: Code number 571.3.

Step 1. Look for the code number, not the page number, in volume 1.

Step 2. Notice the wording "571.3 Alcoholic Liver Damage, unspecified."

　—The code and its title refer to any liver damage caused by alcoholism, without specification as to the nature of the disorder.

　—Since there are no exclusion notes, this is the correct code.

　—If there were an exclusion note, the proper code would be indicated, and this code should again be checked in the numerical list.

Example B: The patient's diagnosis is dyspepsia and heartburn, code number 536.8.

Step 1. Look for the code number in volume 1, the alphabetical index.

Step 2. Notice that there is an exclusion note for heartburn, indicating the code number 787.1. You would need to use two diagnosis codes for this description: 536.8 for dyspepsia and 787.1 for heartburn.

Step 3. Be sure to check code 787.1 in the numerical list for any notes.

Now that you have an idea of how simple diagnosis coding is, make sure you read all of the instructions in the front of the diagnosis book before beginning.

Chapter 11

Procedure Coding

In addition to categorizing patients by diagnosis, physicians like to be reimbursed for procedures, services, supplies, and time spent with each patient. Diagnosis coding does not apply to these items. Instead, payers recognize a five-digit code and modifier.

Current Procedural Terminology, or CPT, is a simplified book that contains this coding and reporting system. According to the American Medical Association (AMA) website, CPT is a registered trademark of the AMA and the most widely accepted medical nomenclature used to report medical procedures and services under public and private health insurance programs. The AMA is a good place to contact to purchase this book. You could also shop at other vendors; just make sure you purchase the current version. Since the CPT is essential to medical billing, it is important to purchase an updated book every year.

The front of the book gives detailed instructions on to how to use the book. You can train yourself using the examples provided. I recommend that you read and don't stop reading until you completely understand it.

Selecting the code that most closely matches the description of the procedure, service, supply, or time spent means the physician will get the highest rate of reimbursement from the payer, and the time it takes to get reimburse could be reduced. Accuracy is most important. Speed will come later.

Start the procedure coding process with the index. The names of procedures and services are listed in alphabetical order. There is a five-digit code next to each name. After locating the code, look up its description in the main portion of the book to verify that you have chosen the one that best describes the service or procedure performed.

In the appendix is a list of modifiers. Look up and read each modifier in case one applies to your procedure or service. You may need to add a modifier to the code you have selected. The CPT explains the usage of modifiers.

Most of the time, the physician has already done the work for you, giving you the code, modifier, and fee to submit to the insurance company. I recommend verifying that the code is current. Everyone makes mistakes, and doctors aren't always up to date with administrative changes. If the code isn't current, I recommend billing with the current code and giving the physician the current code as well.

At times, physicians use a new procedure or service. In that instance, I would locate the code and then check with the physician to confirm that this was the best code to use.

Ask the physician to provide the code, modifier and fee in the paperwork you receive, so you don't have to guess at what the physician meant in the description. The physician usually knows what to charge. If not, a good way to find out is to call several physicians in the same type of practice in the same area and find out what they are charging. Come up with an average of what everyone else is charging.

A great tool to use along with the CPT is a medical dictionary. If the physician's wording differs from the words available in the index of the CPT, you can get other words to try by looking up the description in the dictionary. Referring to the dictionary is also a good way to learn what the description means.

Here is an example of what you might come across when coding a procedure for a physician who is an orthopedic surgeon:

> Description: Open reduction, internal placement screw fixation, comminuted butterfly spiral distal third, humerus fracture, left arm.

Let's assume you don't know anything about orthopedics or coding procedures. The best way to start is by looking up the first word, then the second, and so on.

If you look up *open*, you won't find anything. Move on to *reduction*. You'll find a list, but none apply. Move on to *internal*. Nothing there. Move on to *placement*. The list shows nothing that applies. Move on to *screw*. Nothing there. Move on to *fixation*. You'll see "fixation (device)," but nothing applies.

Then move on to *fracture*, where there are several listings. Look for *humerus*, see *shaft*, and then see *open treatment*. There is a range of codes (24515–24516).

It took a while. But now that you have learned where to find any procedure containing the word *fracture*, you'll save time by going straight to *fracture*, finding the area, and then finding the code. This is a good way to learn from scratch.

Once you've found it, always look up the code—in this case, 24515. This code best describes the description of the procedure. The "butterfly spiral" is unusual and requires unusual work by the physician.

The modifier "22" is also needed with this procedure code. The modifier allows the physician to charge more than what would normally be reimbursed for the procedure code 24515. Find modifiers in the appendix. The code 24515-22 best describes and specifies what the physician performed.

Every time you look up procedures, you learn, so the next time is easier. This is exactly how I learned. I concentrated on accuracy. Speed and knowledge came later.

Now that you know how simple procedure coding can be, make sure you read all of the instructions in the front and throughout the procedure coding book.

Chapter 12

Insurance Coverage Eligibility

As a courtesy to the patient, most physicians bill the patient's insurance. The patient submits a copy of his or her insurance card. In some cases, there is more than one insurance policy that applies; therefore, you need a copy of each insurance card. Make a copy of both sides of the card(s).

Most likely, the physician's office staff will have verified insurance eligibility for each patient before rendering services. It is best to get a copy of this verification when the charges are picked up, because you may need to refer back to the verification if a claim is not paid.

Even though the physician's office may have verified the coverage, it is best that you understand the process. Simply look at the copy of both sides of the patient's insurance card. Usually, the back or lower area of the card will provide a phone number to call in order to verify the patient's eligibility for insurance coverage. If there is no coverage, the physician's fee becomes a debt payable by the patient or guarantor.

CHAPTER 13

Important Items from the Provider

To accurately provide complete billing services for a physician, the physician must provide you with this information:

- Physician's state license number
- Physician's social security number
- Physician's tax identification number
- Patient demographic information, such as name, address, phone number, date of birth, gender, social security number, insurance information, subscriber information, guarantor information, family names, and spouse's name
- Procedure information
- Surgery reports
- Consultation reports
- Diagnosis information
- Assignment of benefits
- Detailed aging report of old patient accounts with outstanding balances
- Letter from the physician stating that your business will be submitting claims on the physician's behalf

Many offices use a universal claim form called the HCFA 1500 for billing insurance companies. Office supply companies—for instance, Office Depot—have these forms available for purchase.

Some payers require a different form. For instance, Medicare and Medicaid require electronic billing. Worker's compensation requires a Doctor's First Report. You must call each insurance company you need to deal with and ask questions about what they require to get the claim paid. Many insurance companies now offer the capability to bill electronically.

Integrated Medical Services is a company that can help you get online for electronic billing. Medisoft is another company offering medical billing software that helps you complete the HCFA 1500 forms as well as online electronic billing. I am sure there are many more companies out there that are competitive for your business. All you have to do is the research to find the most affordable start for your practice.

—♦—

Part Three:

MANAGING YOUR BUSINESS

—♦—

CHAPTER 14

Office Equipment and Supplies List

Computer with backup technology
Word processor program
Excel computer program
Printer
Fax machine
Designated telephone line (with multiple lines if possible)
Answering machine or answering service
File cabinet
Filing system
Copy paper
HCFA 1500 forms
Copy machine
Paper scanner
Filing folders
Labels
Stapler with staples
Pens and pencils
Envelopes
Stamps

CHAPTER 15
Scheduling Yourself

The logistics of obtaining the information you need to bill payers—patient demographics, insurance, procedure (s) performed, fees and diagnoses—depends upon a discussion between you and your client physician. Coordinate your schedules to arrange how you will be picking up charges each week.

The arrangement I usually made was to go on Fridays, because the week was winding down for the physicians and their staff. I would use that day to make all my rounds and pick up the necessary paperwork from each physician. I called the staff in advance to make sure that the paperwork was ready in my pickup spot. That way, all I had to do was walk in, gather my paperwork from the box, and walk out. I was not taking time away from the staff or myself.

Upon returning to my office, I would quickly organize the paperwork by doctor and alphabetize the patients. I logged the doctor's name and the date in my files. Then I listed the patient's name, account number, date of service, amount of the charges, and diagnosis. This way I had my own log of which doctors I had picked up from and which patients were included, in order to refer back to it if I needed to.

Sometimes the office staff would forget to make my copies and give them to me. Later they would call me to see if I had received the charges. I would simply look at my log sheet by doctor and by date to see if I had received those charges. If I had not, I would request my copies. This helped me to stay efficient.

CHAPTER 16

Preparing the Charts

For every patient you will be billing for, you need a filing system that helps you stay accurate and keeps you on track for submitting claims and following up to make sure payment is completed.

I have found that using manila folders with labels for patients' names, like a patient chart in the doctor's office, was cheap and served the purpose. I filed each patient chart by alphabetical order under the name of the treating physician. Organize the chart in such a way that when you open it, you can see what the last completed task was and what needs to happen next.

In my charts, I stored a sheet of paper that I had ruled with columns. The column headers contained places for date of service, charge amount, how paid, payment amount, adjustment amount, total balance, and follow-up made. I stapled this sheet inside the front cover of the patient folder. Every time I filed the claim forms, explanation of benefits from the insurance company, received a charge, received a payment, had to make an adjustment, or any other activity on that account, I made a note on that inside sheet. At a glance, I could see how much the patient's balance was and what other activity had been done. This way, when it came time to go over the aging accounts, I could see if any activity had been done that month on that account.

Steps like these help you stay organized and thorough. Again, this is your business. Any system you choose is appropriate as long as you use it consistently.

CHAPTER 17

Submitting the Charges

Submitting charges to payers in a timely manner is important. Being accurate when submitting those charges is even more important.

Using your computer software, enter all of the data necessary for the mandatory fields on the billing form. In order to know which fields are mandatory, it is important to review the proper way to fill out the HCFA1500 form. There is an interactive web page that allows you to click on the field and learn what information needs to be filled in. The page can be found on the Palmetto GBA website at http://www.palmettogba.com/internet/cms1500.nsf/index.html#. Additional information can be found at the government's Centers for Medicare & Medicaid Services site.

Look through your alphabetized charges to make sure you have each procedure coded and each diagnosis coded.

Make sure all of the patient information and insurance information is there.

An assignment of benefits form signed by the patient allows the insurance company to pay the physician directly. This prevents insurance payments from going to the patient rather than the physician. Make sure each patient has one of these.

Refer to your billing program for details about how to use the software and set up your printer to print the completed HCFA 1500 forms for mailing.

If you are able to submit claims electronically, this is the more efficient and effective method of medical billing. It avoids the task of folding and stuffing envelopes to mail.

Your computer billing software should keep track of patients you have billed. It should allow you to print an accounts receivable report that shows a detailed listing of each account that has a balance, and to separate those balances into charges that are thirty, sixty, ninety, and more days old. Using this report will help you know how the accounts are aging and whether they need to be followed up on. The physician you are billing for may require you to submit this report each month.

Month-End Duties

Each month it is a good practice to send monthly statements to the patients. I sent statements on the last day of the month. Some medical billers send statements for the first half of the patient list on the 15th of every month and the second half of the patient list on the last day of the month. Whatever your preference, just be consistent.

Follow up each month on aging accounts and bill, resubmit, or make adjustments appropriately.

Each month your client physician is likely to require you to submit reports. Include in your proposal a reference to the reports you are willing to provide. (You may recall that my proposal promised the following: "Within ten days after your month-end closing, you will receive a general ledger report that will contain all of the charges billed, the payment adjustments, and the amount of payments deposited during the month. You will also receive a computer-generated report of your total accounts receivable that will tell you how each account is aging. At that time, I will prepare your statement based on_____.")

You must provide any documents you have promised. Additional reporting may be negotiated by the client physician. The timing of these reports will likewise be determined by the agreement between you and the physician. Be thorough and consistent.

The month-end closing includes totals for all charges billed, payments posted, and adjustments posted. These totals should match the list of totals you calculated. Balancing these numbers every month will help you stay accurate.

CHAPTER 19

Billing Follow-Up

Once a bill is submitted to the insurance company, the insurance company has ninety days to pay or deny it. Follow-up on unpaid submitted claims should be done every thirty days. Follow-up can be in the form of a phone call or submission of a paper claim inquiry.

If you decide to follow up with a phone call, always log the date, time, and name of who you spoke with in the patient file, along with the details of the conversation.

If you decide to follow up by submitting a claim inquiry form, it should be printed on your company letterhead. The mailed original should be signed, and a photocopy should be placed in the patient file in case you need to prove that follow-up was done in a timely fashion.

Here is an example of a claim inquiry form that I used. It proved to be effective in a number of situations. Keep in mind that when this letter and the others I will share were developed, I already had several years' experience in billing and collecting. They are informed by many different scenarios you may be encounter while attempting to collect a debt.

Sandra L. Kocsis

****Claim Inquiry****

_____

_____   _____
                                 (date)
_____

(Payer Address)

Patient name_____S.S #_____

Policy #_____ Group #_____ DOS_____

[Reader note: S.S.# = social security number, DOS = date of service]

_____ Payment on this claim is overdue. Please explain the delay.

_____ Please advise as to the status of this claim.

_____ This is the second request for information. Please explain.

_____ Please explain reason for denial.

_____ Only a partial payment was received. Please explain.

_____ An overpayment has occurred. We are returning this money.

_____ We cannot identify this payment. Please send a copy of the claim.

_____ Other:_____
_____

_____ If a check has been issued, please fill out below or send a copy of the canceled check (front and back).

Issued to: _____

Address: _____

Date issued: _____ Amount $ _____

We have billed you as a courtesy to your insured policyholder, who would greatly appreciate your cooperation in paying this claim.

Thank you,

_____

Account Administrator

Let's face it: no one is perfect. You are going to make mistakes. If a claim has been submitted inaccurately, a claim reconsideration form can be submitted with a corrected claim form, as long as the error is found within the ninety-day period from the date of service. Here is an example that I used and found effective. Again, this should be printed on your company letterhead.

Sandra L. Kocsis

****Claim Reconsideration****

_____   _____
_____   (date)
_____
(Payer Address)

Patient name_____S.S #_____

Policy #_____ Group #_____ DOS_____

This claim is being submitted to you for reconsideration of payment. These services were performed for our patient in the best interest of his/her health. Your insured believed this to be a benefit under the patient's policy. Thank you for your help in processing this claim for payment.

Please consider the following reason(s) for reconsideration:

_____ A corrected billing is attached.
_____ A report or documentation is attached.
_____ An Explanation of Benefits (EOB) from the other insurer is attached.
_____ Information you requested is attached.
_____ The claim was denied in error.
_____ Only a partial payment was received.
_____ The insured has contacted you and has now asked us to rebill.
_____ Other: _____

We have billed you as a courtesy to your insured policyholder, who would greatly appreciate your cooperation in paying this claim.

Thank you,

_____
Account Administrator

Having documentation as proof of follow-up on a claim is crucial when you are asking the insurance company to determine whether a claim should be paid.

CHAPTER 20
Collections

Sometimes the patient's insurance has paid a portion of the total and left a balance for the patient to pay. At this point, it is best to send computerized monthly statements to the patient. Many times the patient may have secondary insurance that will pick up the balance, but that information was not obtained by the office staff during the initial visit to the physician.

Here is a sample letter that has proven effective. I sent this to the patient after the insurer paid, sent notification, or both. This letter should be sent *in addition to* a computerized monthly statement.

_____   _____
_____   (date)
_____

(Patient's name and address)

Dear [Patient Name],

As a courtesy to you, we have billed your insurance company
for services rendered to you by Dr. _____ on
_____ for the amount of $_____.
We have received payment/notification, and the balance due of $
_____ is your responsibility;

_____ This is the balance remaining after your insurance has paid.
_____ Charges were applied toward your deductible.
_____ Your insurance company denied benefits.
_____ Your insurance coverage was terminated as of _____.
_____ If you have a secondary insurance company that you would
like billed, please complete:

    Company name_____
    Billing address _____
    Subscriber's name _____
    Policy # _____ Group #_____

_____ Other:_____

_____

Account Administrator

After this initial notification of a balance owed goes out to the patient, follow-up must continue every thirty days or sooner. If you have not heard back from the patient, send a second letter. Remember, sign the original and keep a photocopy in the patient's chart for reference later on.

Here is a letter that I would send to the patient for the secondary follow-up. I would enclose a self-addressed stamped envelope to make it convenient for the patient to send payment right away. This letter has proven effective.

_____   _____
                                              (date)
_____

_____

(Patient's name and address)

Dear [Patient Name],

This is the *second* request for payment on the balance of
$_____ remaining on your account. This is for services
rendered to you some time ago by Dr. _____.

_____ This is the balance after your insurance has paid.

_____ This is the balance after both insurances have paid.

_____ Your insurance was billed but denied benefits.

_____ Computerized monthly statements have been sent to you.

_____ See attached copies of manual billings sent to you.

_____ The phone number we have for you is not current.

_____ Other: _____

If this has already been paid, please send us a copy of your canceled
check or explanation of benefits from your insurance carrier, and
we are sorry for your inconvenience.

If this hasn't been paid, we would appreciate your help in finally
clearing this balance. Please give us a call at _____
if you have any questions regarding your account. A self-addressed,
stamped envelope is enclosed for your convenience.

Thank you,

_____

Account Administrator

If settlement on the patient's account balance has not been resolved within thirty days of the secondary follow-up, then a third letter to request payment must be sent. This letter is sent in addition to the monthly computerized statements you have been sending all along. This letter has proven effective.

———————————   ———————————
———————————   (date)
———————————

(Patient's name and address)

Dear [Patient Name],

This is the *third* request for payment on the balance of $———————————remaining on your account. This is for services rendered to you some time ago by Dr. ———————————.

We would really like to make suitable arrangements for payment.

If we do not hear from you within ten days from the date on this letter, formal collection proceedings will begin.

If this balance has already been paid, please send us a copy of your canceled check or explanation of benefits from your insurance carrier, and we are sorry for your inconvenience.

If this hasn't been paid, we would appreciate your help in finally clearing this balance. Please give us a call at ———————————
if you have any questions regarding your account. A self-addressed, stamped envelope is enclosed for your convenience.

Thank you,

———————————————————

Account Administrator

P.S. Please send all payments to the address on the letterhead above.

If the patient or guarantor does not contact you to make payment arrangements within the ten days stipulated, you will need to send a fourth letter. In the meantime, you need to be thinking about next steps.

Communicate with the physician about your attempts to collect and ask the physician how he or she would like to proceed. Often these accounts can be submitted to an outside collection agency, taken to court for a judgment or a lien on the patient's assets, or written off as a bad debt. In other cases, the physician may ask you to continue your collection efforts or to write off the balance. This is strictly up to the physician for whom you are collecting.

Whatever the decision, you need to make sure you follow through with what you said you were going to do. This sample fourth letter is one I used when the decision has been made to move on to formal collection proceedings.

_____   _____
_____   (date)
_____
(Patient's name and address)

Dear Patient,

As the result of *no response* for payment arrangements on your remaining account balance of $_____, you will be reported to the credit bureaus and judicial proceedings will be instituted. This is for services rendered to you some time ago by Dr._____.

You can stop these actions by giving us a call. We will work with you and are looking forward to hearing from you.

If this balance has already been paid, please send us a copy of your canceled check or explanation of benefits from your insurance carrier, and we are sorry for your inconvenience.

If this hasn't been paid, we would appreciate your help in finally clearing this balance. Please give us a call at _____ if you have any questions regarding your account. A self-addressed, stamped envelope is enclosed for your convenience.

Thank you,

_____
Account Administrator

Sometimes patient account balances become overlooked, and the only action you have taken has been sending monthly statements. In that case, when the patient's account has become older than ninety days or if you are trying to act as the collection agency, you can send this letter to the patient. This letter could act as the first letter and the beginning of your collection efforts. This letter has proven effective.

_____   _____

_____   (date)

_____

(Patient's name and address)

Dear [Patient Name],

As the result of a recent audit, your account has been sent to me for collection. We have noticed a balance of $_____ remaining on your account. This is for services rendered to you some time ago by Dr. _____.

_____ This is the balance after your insurance has paid.
_____ This is the balance after both insurances have paid.
_____ Your insurance was billed but denied benefits.
_____ Computerized monthly statements have been sent to you.
_____ See attached copies of manual billings sent to you.
_____ The phone number we have for you is not current.
_____ Other: _____

If this has already been paid, please send us a copy of your canceled check or explanation of benefits from your insurance carrier, and we are sorry for your inconvenience.

If this hasn't been paid, we would appreciate your help in finally clearing this balance. Please give us a call at_____ if you have any questions regarding your account. A self-addressed, stamped envelope is enclosed for your convenience.

Thank you,

_____

Account Administrator

Consider giving patients the best possible chance to resolve their financial issues. These letters and processes help with that. Having patience and being consistent usually result in the patient making payment arrangements. I have only been to court one time on a debt that the surgeon really wanted collected.

When your collection efforts land you at a point of decision, consider whether the physician will take a partial payment and write off the rest. That way, all is not lost.

For every patient that I performed follow-up on, I kept a list by month that had the doctor's name, patient account number, last name of the patient, what transpired, and amount of the claim. This way, when the physician wanted to know what my efforts had been to collect on the debt, I could show him or her immediately.

When I was able to collect a debt in full or partially, I kept a payment/adjustment sheet. This sheet had the doctor's name, date, patient's account number, patient's name, date of service being paid/adjusted, payment type (cash, insurance, check, Medicare, Medicaid), adjustment type (charge/data, bad debt, payment adjustment required by insurance, or an insurance-only agreement on the account), and the dollar amount of the payment/adjustment.

Every payment and adjustment should be entered into the patient's account on your computer, using your medical billing program. This will show up on the printed statements that are sent to the physician each month.

I only billed the physician my percentage on the amount of the payment, not on the original billed amount.

Chapter 21

Billing Your Fee

Determining what you will charge the physicians is up to you. Some medical billers charge a fixed fee per line item. Some charge a percentage of the total amount billed.

Personally, I charged 7 percent of what I collected, not what I billed. I determined this percentage by calling all of the billing services in my area and obtaining an average of what they charged—then I reduced that charge by half. My thinking was that my overhead was half that of a business that leased or bought a building. Plus, I was doing all of my own work and had no employees. I believe this advantageous billing rate helped physicians determine whether they would hire me as their account representative. Again, it is your business, and you can determine the fee structure that works for you.

To invoice my clients at the end of the month, I created a statement of collections. I calculated the amount that I had collected, deducted my 7 percent, and showed that the net amount of collections had been deposited in the physician's account. Showing the math demonstrated that I was accurate. If there were any balances that did not match, I did not close the month's end until I balanced to the penny. This kept me on track and showed my clients that I focused on accuracy.

Conclusion

When I set out to write this book, I knew that I had some information and ideas that could help others get started. I had gotten my start with a desire to work for myself, and that desire turned into ambition.

I could not have done this alone. I want to thank all the people out there who helped me and who believed in me. It takes guts to trust someone you don't know to do the billing and collections for your medical practice. Private information was entrusted to me, and my clients showed me faith that I would only use that information for its proper purpose.

As I mentioned, running your own business takes work. Preparation is the key to ensuring a smooth transition when taking over a physician's billing. You are not alone. There is a wealth of information out there to help you. The information I have provided will make that transition run more smoothly.

Remember that this is your business, and it is up to you to make sure that your office and its systems are ready for use. The bottom line here is that you really have to want to start your own home-based medical billing service. You have to see yourself actually doing it. Be confident. Act as if you are doing it, never give up, and eventually you will be doing it.

My hope is that you understand that if I can do it, so can you.

Additional Resources

The Affordable Care Act, also called Obamacare, is described in detail at the Health and Human Services website at http://www.hhs.gov/.

The American Medical Association provides information and products related to physician practices, medical ethics, medical billing, and more at http://www.ama-assn.org/ama.

The California Department of Health Care Services handles one of the biggest state-run insurance programs in the country, Medi-Cal. Learn more at http://www.dhcs.ca.gov/Pages/default.aspx.

The Center for Medicare & Medicaid Services offers an abundance of information on their Web site including a Medicare claims processing manual, at http://www.cms.gov/Regulations-and-Guidance/Guidance/Manuals/Downloads/clm104c26.pdf.

EDS is a software company whose products are used by payers and billers. You can view one of their user manuals at http://www.vtmedicaid.com/Downloads/software/PES%20User%20Guide%20507.pdf.

Guffey, M. E. (2009). *Essentials of business communication* (8th ed.). Mason, Ohio: South-Western Cengage Learning.

HIPAA is described in detail at the Health and Human Services website at http://www.hhs.gov/ocr/privacy/.

The Internal Revenue Service provides all of its forms and information booklets online at http://www.irs.gov/.

Lewis, S. (2013). *Medical-surgical nursing* (8th ed.). St. Louis, Missouri: Elsevier Mosby.

Medisoft is a medical software program published by McKesson. You can learn more about it at their website http://www.medisoft.com/.

Morrison, E. (2011). *Ethics in health administration: A practical approach for decision makers* (2nd ed.). London, UK: Jones and Bartlett Publishers.

Nix, K. (2011, January 10). The impact of Obamacare: From the frontlines of our healthcare crisis. Retrieved from http://blog.heritage.org/2011/01/10/the-impact-of-obamacare-from-the-frontlines-of-our-health-care-crisis/.

Optum Coding sells coding manuals, medical billing software, and training at https://www.optumcoding.com.

OWL: The Online Writing Lab at Purdue University is an excellent resource to enhance your writing skills, providing information, samples, and exercises at https://owl.english.purdue.edu/.

The Small Business Administration, a federal program, provides information and services to help you start, grow, and succeed in your small business at http://www.sbaonline.sba.gov/.

About the Author

Sandra Kocsis is the mother of three very precious daughters, Ashley, Dani, and Amy. She has spent her entire career in the medical field, beginning as a clerk for a medical billing service in 1987 and progressing through office management to become an instructor at a vocational college, where she taught front office skills, billing and collections, how to take vital signs, and medical terminology. She always encouraged her students to set out on their own. Then it occurred to her that she should take her own advice. Now she wants to help others who are willing to tackle the work-from-home adventure.

www.ingramcontent.com/pod-product-compliance
Lightning Source LLC
Chambersburg PA
CBHW030915180526
45163CB00004B/1848